D0891677

CALLISTA ROY

Notes on Nursing Theories

SERIES EDITORS

Chris Metzger McQuiston
Private Practice

Adele A. Webb
College of Nursing, University of Akron

The purpose of this series of monographs is to provide the reader with a concise description of conceptual frameworks and theories in nursing. It is not intended to replace the primary works of nurse theorists, but to provide direction for their use. Designed for undergraduate students, these monographs will also be helpful guides for graduate students and faculty.

Due to the complexity of existing books and chapters on nursing conceptual frameworks and theories, students often have difficulty understanding and incorporating nursing theory into their practice. The concise monographs of this series include a biographical sketch of the theorist, origin of the theory, assumptions, concepts, propositions, examples for application to practice and research, glossary of terms, and a bibliography of classic works, critiques, and research. Organization of the information in this manner will facilitate student understanding and use, thereby broadening the base of nursing science.

Volume 1
Martha Rogers: The Science of Unitary Human Beings
Louette R. Johnson Lutjens

Volume 2
Imogene King: A Conceptual Framework for Nursing
Christina L. Sieloff Evans

Volume 3
Callista Roy: An Adaptation Model
Louette R. Johnson Lutjens

Volume 4
Dorothea Orem: Self-Care Deficit Theory
Donna L. Hartweg

CALLISTA ROY

An Adaptation Model

Louette R. Johnson Lutjens

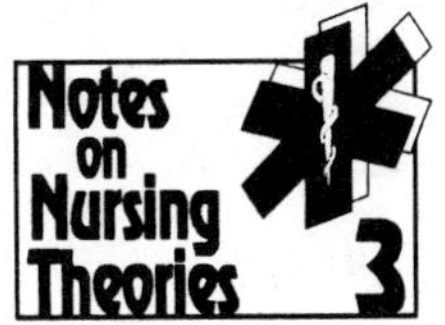

SAGE PUBLICATIONS
The International Professional Publishers
Newbury Park London New Delhi

For information address:

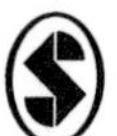

SAGE Publications, Inc.
2455 Teller Road
Newbury Park, California 91320

SAGE Publications Ltd.
6 Bonhill Street
London EC2A 4PU
United Kingdom

SAGE Publications India Pvt. Ltd.
M-32 Market
Greater Kailash I
New Delhi 110 048 India

Printed in the United States of America

Library of Congress Cataloging-in-Publication Data

Lutjens, Louette R. Johnson
Callista Roy : an adaptation model / Louette R. Johnson Lutjens.
p. cm. — (Notes on nursing theories : v. 3)
Includes bibliographical references.
ISBN 0-8039-4228-1 (cl) ISBN 0-8039-4228-1 (pb)
1. Nursing — Philosophy. 2. Nursing. I. Title II. Series.
RT84.5.L88 1991
610.73'01—dc20 91-29792
CIP

FIRST PRINTING, 1991

Sage Production Editor: Michelle R. Starika

To my parents,
Catherine A. Nesbit Johnson and W. Peter Johnson, and
my parents-in-law,
E. Jane Weissenberger and Edwin Weissenberger

Contents

Foreword

When you walk onto our unit at Montefiore Medical Center you often will not see a nurse. The nurses are with the patients and their families. Since the implementation of the Roy Adaptation Model for theory based practice, there is a new perspective of the nurse-patient relationship.

The evolution of nursing models has been rapid. Over the last five years, the development of nursing theory derived from these models has also grown dramatically, adding to the scientific base of nursing. Because nursing is a practice discipline, the ultimate goal of nursing theory is to guide and enhance that practice.

Each of the nursing models and related theories provides a particular lens for the nurse to use when viewing nursing situations. The Roy Adaptation Model provides one of these lenses. Roy's view of the person as an adaptive system is a particularly useful one given the complex nature of the problems nurses encounter in today's heath care arena.

The value of the Roy Model is in its ability to serve as a framework for practice, education, administration, and research. Dr. Louette Lutjens has masterfully presented the model in a way that emphasizes its value for contributing to each of these areas. She also demonstrates how the Roy Adaptation Model provides a viable framework for organizing and providing nursing care as well as for building nursing knowledge through theory development.

As nursing educators increasingly include nursing models in the beginning education levels of the profession, as well as in graduate studies, nurses will increasingly depend on nursing conceptual models in their practice. The utilization of monographs such as this will serve nursing well by providing a guide for nurses to make informed and assertive demands for theory based practice.

Through this monograph, Dr. Lutjens offers the next generation of nurses an enhanced pride of membership in a truly scientific profession.

KEVILLE FREDERICKSON, RN, EDD
Professor of Nursing,
Lehman College of the City University
of New York, and Clinical Nurse Scientist,
Montefiore Medical Center
Bronx, NY

Preface

The nursing profession is fortunate to have many nurse theorists who have provided the discipline with conceptual models with which to view the world of nursing. The various models capture the diversity inherent in nursing while at the same time shaping its unique body of knowledge.

Sister Dr. Callista Roy is a well-known nurse theorist whose conceptual model is based on the concept of adaptation. This volume presents a current, succinct description of the Roy Adaptation Model, as well as the theory of Person as an Adaptive System and the Theory of Adaptive Modes. Serving as a summary of the basic concepts of the model and derived theories, this volume supplements the original primary sources primarily Roy and Roberts (1981), Roy (1984), Andrews and Roy (1986), and Roy and Andrews (1991).

This volume is intended primarily for undergraduate students who are studying several nursing models with their differing terms, language, and theory-specific definitions of common concepts. It could also be used as a brief review by nursing faculty and graduate students.

A bibliography is provided to direct readers to appropriate sources for in-depth information on the Roy model, including use of the nursing process, applications to practice and education, and analysis and critique of the conceptual model. It is hoped that this description of the Roy Adaptation Model will entice readers to make use of the references provided.

I would like to acknowledge the careful and thoughtful critique of this text by Dr. Patricia Underwood, Associate Professor and Coordinator of the Graduate Program at Kirkhof School of Nursing, Grand Valley State University, Allendale, MI. Dr. Underwood is also the current president of the Michigan Nurses' Association. Also, I would like to thank Sister Callista Roy for her review of an earlier draft of this text and her encouragement and support over the past several years.

—LOUETTE R. JOHNSON LUTJENS

Biographical Sketch of a Nurse Theorist: Sister Callista Roy, PhD, RN, FAAN

Born: October 14, 1939
BA: Nursing, Mount St. Mary's College, Los Angeles, 1963
MSN: University of California, Los Angeles, 1966
MA: Sociology, University of California, Los Angeles, 1975
PhD: Sociology, University of California, Los Angeles, 1977
Post Doctoral Fellow: Robert Wood Johnson Clinical Nurse Scholar Program (Neuroscience), University of California, San Francisco, 1983-1985
Fellow: American Academy of Nursing
Member: Sisters of St. Joseph of Carondolet
Position: Professor, School of Nursing, Boston College

1

Origin of the Model

While a graduate student at the University of California, Los Angeles (1964-1966), Sister Dr. Callista Roy was challenged in a seminar by another nurse theorist, Dorothy E. Johnson, to develop a theory of nursing. Subsequently, in 1964, the Roy Adaptation Model (RAM) was born as a derivation of Bertalanffy's General Systems Theory and Harry Helson's Adaptation-Level Theory. Other experts in the field of adaptation who influenced Roy in the development of her model included Dohrenwend, Lazarus, Mechanic, and Selye. Rapoport's ideas in the area of systems and Maslow's thoughts on human needs also contributed to the model.

The adaptation concept was introduced to Roy in a psychology class. In her clinical work in pediatric nursing, she had been impressed with the ability of children to bounce back when faced with illness. The adaptation concept seemed to be a suitable concept upon which to base a conceptual model of nursing. Roy's ultimate goal was "to demonstrate that the practice of nursing, based on the science of nursing, makes a difference in the health status of the population" (Roy & Roberts, 1981, xv). Roy estimates that more than 1,500 faculty and students have contributed to the theoretical development of the Roy Model (Andrews & Roy, 1991a).

The Roy Adaptation Model was first formally utilized in 1968 as the conceptual framework for the baccalaureate nursing curriculum at Mount St. Mary's College in Los Angeles, where Roy was chairperson of the Department of Nursing. Roy is a prolific writer who has spent much time and effort over the years developing and refining the model. The seminal and classic theory text on the Roy Adaptation Model is *Theory Construction in Nursing: An Adaptation Model* written by Roy and Sharon Roberts and published in 1981. Roy works extremely well with other nurse scholars on a national and international basis, mentoring them in the use of her model in education, service, practice, and research. Roy's contributions to nursing science are commendable and significant.

2

Assumptions of the Model

Assumptions are "givens"—that is, statements assumed to be true without proof. With any conceptual model or theory, students must be able to accept the assumptions before adopting the specific model or theory.

Scientific Assumptions

Roy's scientific assumptions have received much attention in the literature. These eight assumptions, which are based on systems and adaptation-level theories, are as follows:

1. The person is a bio-psycho-social being.
2. The person is in constant interaction with a changing environment.
3. To cope with a changing world, the person uses both innate and acquired mechanisms, which are biologic, psychologic, and social in origin.
4. Health and illness are one inevitable dimension of life.
5. To respond positively to environmental changes, the person must adapt.
6. The person's adaptation is a function of the stimulus exposed to and one's adaptation level.

7. The person's adaptation level is such that it comprises a zone that indicates the range of stimulation that will lead to a positive response.
8. The person is conceptualized as having four modes of adaptation: physiologic, self-concept, role function, and interdependence. (Roy, 1980, pp. 180-182)[1]

Philosophical Assumptions

Until recently, the philosophical assumptions of the RAM had not been as explicit, specific, and organized as the scientific assumptions. Roy (1988) addressed this limitation by a thoughtful explication of eight philosophical assumptions, four based on the philosophical principle of humanism and four based on the philosophical principle of "veritivity" (a word coined by Roy).

Humanism. Humanism "recognizes the person and subjective dimensions of human experience as central to knowing and to valuing" (Roy, 1988, p. 29). Roy credits Maslow with influencing her thoughts on humanism. The four philosophical assumptions based on the humanist principle are as follows:

1. The individual shares in creative power,
2. Behaves purposefully, not in a sequence of cause and effect,
3. Possesses intrinsic holism, and
4. Strives to maintain integrity and to realize the need for relationships.

Veritivity. The term *veritivity,* derived from the Latin *veritas,* meaning truth, was coined by Roy. The premise underlying Roy's term is that there is an absolute truth. Roy (1988) defines veritivity "as a principle of human nature that affirms a common purposefulness of human existence" (p. 30). The four philosophical assumptions based on the veritivity principle are as follows:

1. The individual is viewed in the context of the purposefulness of human existence,
2. Unity of purpose of humankind,

3. Activity and creativity for the common good, and
4. Value and meaning of life. (p. 32)

The eight scientific and eight philosophical assumptions provide a basis for theorizing and research within the RAM.

Note

1. Slight revisions have been made in the scientific assumptions to reflect changes made by Roy over the years.

3

Concepts of the Model

Roy's model is a systems model that focuses on outcomes. The major features of systems models are the system and its environment. According to Andrews and Roy (1991a), "a system is a set of parts connected to function as a whole for some purpose and does so by virtue of the interdependence of its parts" (p. 7). A system is open, nonmechanistic; behavior is determined by the free interplay of changing forces (Roy & Anway, 1989).

Roy views adaptation as both a process and a product or end-state. The process of adaptation is described as one in which stressors produce, at least in part, an interaction called stress. Stress triggers the use of coping behaviors to assist persons to reduce or alleviate the stress. The ways or methods of coping produce adaptive or ineffective responses. Adaptation is a process that "involves a systematic series of actions directed toward some end" (Roy, 1990). The result of the process of adaptation is the end-state or outcome of adaptation. Adaptation as a state is "the condition of the person with respect to the environment" (Roy, 1990).

In the Roy Adaptation Model, the person is conceptualized as an open adaptive system engaging in interchange with the environment. Roy and McLeod (1981) described adaptation for the open system of an individual as "the person's response to the environment which promotes the general goals of the person including survival, growth, reproduction, and mastery" (p. 53). Major factors influencing the adaptation of the person throughout life are culture, family, and growth and development (Sato, 1984).

Person

Key concepts in the Roy Adaptation Model are person, goal, health, environment, and nursing activities. Roy uses person in her model as a concept to identify the recipient of nursing care. Critical to the model is the description of recipients of nursing care as holistic adaptive systems. The term *adaptive* "means that the human system has the capacity to adjust effectively to changes in the environment and, in turn, affect the environment" (Andrews & Roy, 1991a, p. 7). Persons employ coping mechanisms to assist them in adapting to their environment. Roy has identified four major areas in which the activities of the coping mechanisms can be seen. She refers to these areas as adaptive modes. Together, the coping mechanisms and the modes reflect the integration of the individual.

Goal

The goal of nursing within this model is to promote adaptation in four adaptive modes (physiologic, self-concept, role function, and interdependence) and thereby contribute to health. When people are in an adaptive state, they are free to respond to other stimuli. "This freeing of energy links the concept of adaptation to the concept of health" (Roy, 1984, p. 38).

Health

Health has been defined as "a state and a process of being and becoming an integrated and whole person" (Andrews & Roy, 1991a, p. 19). Holism and integrated functioning are not only basic premises of systems theory (Roy & Anway, 1989), but are also congruent with the philosophical assumptions of Roy's model (Roy, 1988).

Health as a state reflects the adaptation process and is demonstrated by adaptation in each of four integrated adaptive modes: physiologic, self-concept, role function, and interdependence. The integration of these four adaptive modes reflects wholeness.

Health is a process whereby individuals are striving to achieve their maximum potential. This process can be readily seen in healthy people who exercise regularly, do not smoke, and pay attention to their dietary habits. The process of health can also be seen in persons in the terminal stages of cancer as they seek control over symptoms, such as pain, and strive for integration within themselves and in relation to significant others.

Environment

Roy has broadly defined environment as "all conditions, circumstances, and influences that surround and affect the development and behavior of the person" (Andrews & Roy, 1991a, p. 18) or group (Roy, 1984, p. 39). Thus all stimuli, whether internal or external, are part of the person's environment. Within her model, Roy specifically categorizes stimuli as focal, contextual, and residual. (The categories of stimuli will be discussed later.) Changes in the environment act as catalysts, stimulating persons to make adaptive responses.

Nursing Activities

The last key concept in the Roy Adaptation Model is nursing activities, which have been described as the nursing process. The nursing process, according to the Roy model, consists of six steps: assessment of behavior, assessment of stimuli, nursing diagnosis, goal setting, intervention, and evaluation. Roy describes two levels of assessment. The first level consists of an assessment of behavior in each of the adaptive modes. Behavior is an indicator of how well persons are adapting to or managing to cope with changes in their health status. Areas of concern or adaptive problems evolve through a mutual (nurse and patient) process in the form of ineffective behaviors needing modification or adaptive behaviors needing reinforcing. An initial tentative nursing judgment is made at this level as to whether the patient behaviors are adaptive or ineffective. Andrews and Roy (1991b) have developed typologies of commonly recurring adaptation problems (pp. 41-42) and indicators of positive adaptation (pp. 38-39) associated with each of the four modes. (Examples of adaptation problems and indicators of positive adaptation will be given in the sections on adaptive modes.)

The second level of assessment involves the identification of focal, contextual, and residual stimuli that have influenced those behaviors that are of concern to the nurse and the patient. Common contextual stimuli that have an effect on behavior in all adaptive modes are culture, family, developmental stage, integrity of adaptive modes, effectiveness of the cognator processes, and other environmental factors, such as the use of drugs, alcohol, and tobacco (Andrews & Roy, 1991b). Nursing diagnoses are made based on the nurse's interpretation of assessment data. The diagnoses are clinical judgments conveying the person's adaptation status that may be stated in one of three ways: as a summary label (e.g., anxiety) for behaviors in one mode (self-concept); as a statement of the behaviors within one mode with the most relevant influencing stimuli (e.g., symptoms of anxiety from medical treatment of cancer); or as a label that summarizes a behavioral pattern when more than one mode is being affected by the same stimuli (e.g., depression related to loss of breast) (Andrews & Roy, 1991b).

Goals are stated in terms of patient outcomes after they have been mutually agreed upon by patient and nurse. Nursing interventions are selected and directed toward the management of stimuli to produce adaptive responses that promote health and well-being. Nursing management is directed toward altering the focal stimulus or broadening the adaptation level by changing the other stimuli present. "When energy is freed from ineffective coping attempts, this energy can promote healing and enhance health" (Roy, 1984, p. 38). The relation-

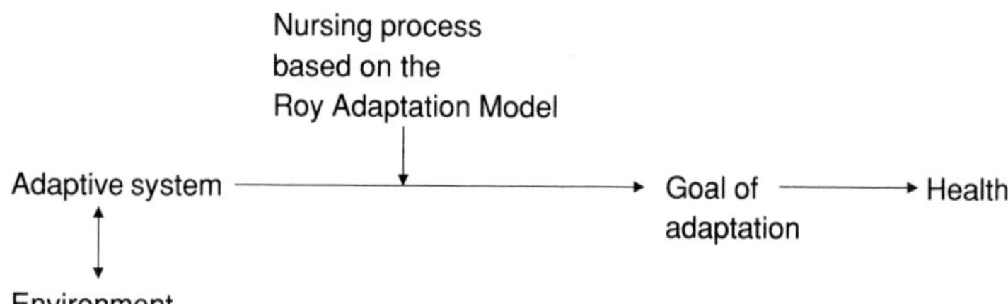

Figure 3.1. Relationships between the key concepts of the Roy model.
SOURCE: Roy, 1984, p. 40. Reprinted by permission.

ships among the major concepts in the Roy Adaptation Model (RAM) are presented in Figure 3.1.

4

Theory of Person as an Adaptive System

In 1981, Roy and McLeod developed a Theory of Person as an Adaptive System from the Roy Adaptation Model. In addition to the concepts of person, goal of nursing, health, environment, and nursing activities in the model, the Theory of Person as an Adaptive System employs additional concepts.

Focal, Contextual, and Residual Stimuli

The Roy Adaptation Model describes the environment as comprising external and internal stimuli that act as stressors. These stimuli serve as input to the person, provoking a response (behavior). The stimuli have been categorized as focal, contextual, and residual. Each of the three categories can include stimuli from external and internal sources. The focal stimulus is the provoking situation or event immediately confronting persons that demands attention and prompts persons to seek relief. Contextual stimuli are all other stimuli present in the situation, or surrounding the event, that contribute to the effect of the focal stimulus. Residual stimuli are those general, vague, ambiguous factors that may be affecting a person, but their influence cannot be immediately ascertained or validated. After residual stimuli are validated, they become either focal or contextual stimuli.

More important than making fine-line distinctions about what to label a stimulus (focal, contextual, residual) is to understand which stimuli are influencing a situation and what individual factors determine how a person perceives and responds to the influencing stimuli. A given factor is not automatically a focal or contextual stimulus. It may be a focal stimulus in one situation and a contextual stimulus in another.

Adaptation Level

Helson first used the term adaptation level to label the combined effect of the three classes of stimuli (focal, contextual, and residual). In addition to the influence of the particular stimuli, the adaptation level, or combination of stimuli, influences the person. Adaptation level is a constantly changing point that represents the person's ability to cope with the changing environment in a positive manner. Adaptation level sets up a zone or range within which stimulation will lead to adaptive responses. Stimuli falling outside this adaptive zone lead to ineffective responses. Suicide due to inability to cope with the death of a child is an extreme example of an ineffective response.

If one accepts that people can be taught coping skills and can learn coping skills from life experiences, then it follows that people can change their own adaptation level to more positively deal with the challenges of everyday life. Thus the person is not passive in relation to the environment. People are active participants interacting with the environment and formulating adaptive responses—those responses contributing to general goals of survival, growth, reproduction, and mastery. Roy views these goals in a broad sense. Growth as a goal is more than an increase in physical size; individuals grow cognitively, psychologically, emotionally, and spiritually. Reproduction as a general goal is viewed as generating or "bringing forth" through a variety of human accomplishments, such as producing a pictorial or literary work of art, in addition to producing children (Roy, 1990).

Coping Mechanisms

Within the process of adaptation, coping refers to the use of behavior in response to stimuli. Defined broadly, coping refers to the use of both routine and nonroutine behaviors (Roy & McLeod, 1981). In a routine sense, coping refers to the use of accustomed patterns of behavior employed by individuals in dealing with daily situations. Roy also uses coping to refer to the use of new behaviors in response to unusual or drastic situations wherein accustomed responses are ineffective. Meeting the challenges of the unexpected allows for creative, novel responses. Inherited (genetically determined) or acquired ways of responding to the changing environment, are referred to as coping mechanisms.

According to Roy, coping mechanisms are of two types: regulator and cognator. The regulator is used primarily as a mechanism to cope with physiological stimuli, while the cognator is used mainly as a mechanism to cope with psychosocial stimuli, dealing primarily in areas of cognition, judgment, and emotion. Regulator and cognator mechanisms are linked through the process of perception. Frequently, the regulator mechanism operates at a level below cognitive awareness. At times, however, outputs from the regulator subsystem are translated into perceptions in the cognator subsystem. While the initial processing of stimuli within the regulator and cognator mechanisms cannot be observed, cognitive perceptions and the behavioral outcomes of these coping mechanisms are amenable to assessment. The behaviors will generally fall into one of four adaptive modes, each contributing to the "promotion of the adaptive goals of the total person system—survival, growth, reproduction, and mastery" (Roy & McLeod, 1981, p. 67).

Adaptive Modes

The concept of adaptive modes did not appear in the literature until 1971. Adaptive modes evolved at the request of students who felt

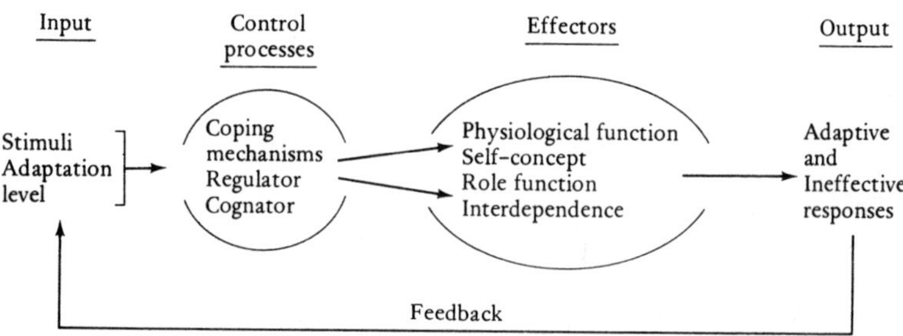

Figure 4.1. The person as an adaptive system.
SOURCE: Roy, 1984, p. 30. Reprinted by permission.

a need for a way to organize assessment data. In 1970, approximately 500 samples of patient behaviors from all clinical areas were collected by baccalaureate nursing students (Roy, 1971). These behaviors were then categorized into what came to be known as adaptive modes. An example of a pediatric history and assessment based on adaptive modes can be found in Andrews and Roy (1986, pp. 173-177).

Roy has identified four adaptive modes: physiological, self-concept, role function, and interdependence. Although these modes will be discussed further under the section on Theory of Adaptive Modes, it is important to recognize that it is the *manifestation* of the coping mechanisms that can be observed and measured within the adaptive modes. Thus the adaptive modes are often referred to as effectors.

Adaptive Responses

Behaviors that contribute to the general goals of persons (i.e., survival, growth, reproduction, and mastery) are considered adaptive responses. Behaviors not contributing to general goals are considered ineffective responses. Adaptive responses bring about a state of adaptation. A diagram depicting the relationships among the concepts of the Theory of Person as an Adaptive System is presented in Figure 4.1.

Propositions

A proposition is a statement about a particular concept or the relationship between concepts. Roy and Roberts (1981) use the term "to describe the initial relationship between variables asserted by the theory" (p. 12). Propositions are important because we can use them to develop hypotheses that can be tested in the clinical area. Roy has developed many propositions from her theories.

Regulator Subsystem Propositions. The first set of propositions is related to the role of the regulator subsystem in the adaptation of persons. The regulator subsystem comprises inputs, major parts, processes, effectors, and feedback loops. Figure 4.2 depicts the regulator subsystem.

Roy's background as a neuroscience post-doctoral fellow is clearly evident in her conceptualization of the regulator subsystem. Inputs consist of external stimuli and internal stimuli from changes in the person's dynamic equilibrium, commonly known as homeostasis. "The inputs are chemical in nature or have been transduced into neural information" (Roy & McLeod, 1981, p. 60). As readers can see from the middle of Figure 4.2, the major parts of the regulator are neural, endocrine, and perception/psychomotor. The propositions that have been developed for the regulator subsystem are related to Figure 4.2 by numbers and are as follows:

- 1.1. Internal and external stimuli are basically chemical or neural; chemical stimuli may be transduced into neural inputs to the central nervous system.
- 1.2. Neural pathways to and from the central nervous system must be intact and functional if neural stimuli are to influence body responses.
- 2.1. Spinal cord, brainstem, and autonomic reflexes act through effectors to produce automatic, unconscious effects on the body responses.
- 3.1. The circulation must be intact for chemical stimuli to influence endocrine glands to produce the appropriate hormone.

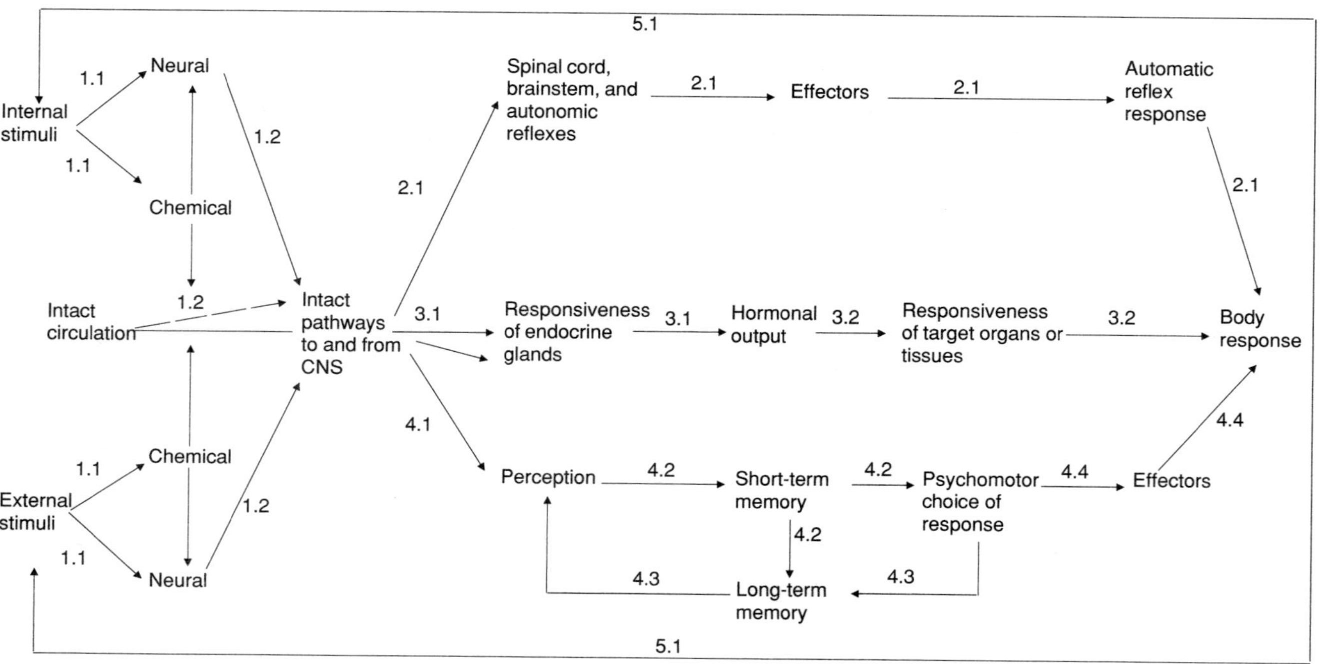

Figure 4.2. The regulator subsystem.
SOURCE: Roy & Roberts, 1981, p. 61. Reprinted by permission.

3.2. Target organs or tissues must be able to respond to hormone levels to effect body responses.

4.1. Neural inputs are transformed into conscious perceptions in the brain (process unknown).

4.2. Increase in short-term or long-term memory will positively influence the effective choice of psychomotor response to neural input.

4.3. Effective choice of response, retained in long-term memory, will facilitate future effective choice of response.

4.4. The psychomotor response chosen will determine the effectors activated and the ultimate body response.

> 1.1 through 2.1, 3.2, 4.4. The magnitude of the internal and external stimuli will positively influence the magnitude of the physiological response of an intact system.
>
> 3.1 through 2.1, 4.4. Intact neural pathways will positively influence neural output to effectors.
>
> 1.1 through 3.2. Chemical and neural inputs will influence normally responsive endocrine glands to hormonally influence target organs in a positive manner to maintain a state of dynamic equilibrium.
>
> 1.1 through 5.1. The body's response to external and internal stimuli will alter those external and internal stimuli.
>
> 1.1 through 5.1. The magnitude of the external and internal stimuli may be so great that the adaptive systems cannot return the body to a state of dynamic equilibrium. (Roy & McLeod, 1981, p. 62)

Cognator Subsystem Propositions. Figure 4.3 depicts the cognator subsystem. A little less complex than the regulator subsystem, the cognator comprises input, parts, processes, and effectors. Inputs are positive and negative internal and external stimuli that include physiological, psychological, social, and spiritual factors. Internal stimuli include the output of the regulator subsystem. Parts consist of apparatus and pathways that enable processes, thereby bringing about a psychomotor choice of response. Effectors are internal and external verbalizations. As with the regulator mechanism, the numbers in the figure correspond to the propositions, which are as follows:

1.1. The optimum amount and clarity of input of internal and external stimuli positively influence the adequacy of selective attention, coding, and memory.

1.2. The optimum amount and clarity of input of internal and external stimuli positively influence the adequacy of imitation, reinforcement, and insight.

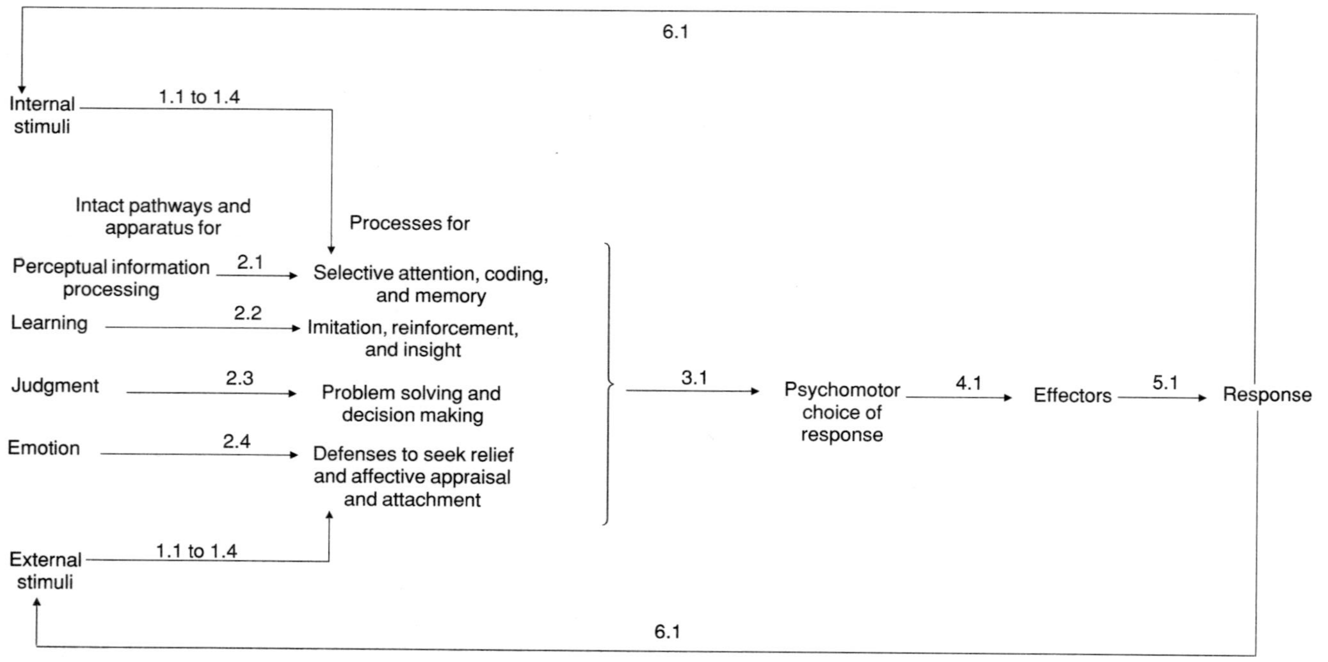

Figure 4.3 The cognator subsystem.

SOURCE: Roy & Roberts, 1981, p. 64. Reprinted by permission.

1.3. The optimum amount and clarity of input of internal and external stimuli positively influence the adequacy of problem solving and decision making.

1.4. The optimum amount and clarity of input of internal and external stimuli positively influence the adequacy of defenses to seek relief, and affective appraisal and attachment.

2.1. Intact pathways and perceptual/information-processing apparatus positively influence the adequacy of selective attention, coding, and memory.

2.2. Intact pathways and learning apparatus positively influence imitation, reinforcement, and insight.

2.3. Intact pathways and judgment apparatus positively influence problem solving and decision making.

2.4. Intact pathways and emotional apparatus positively influence defenses to seek relief, and affective appraisal and attachment.

3.1. The higher the level of adequacy of all the cognator processes, the more effective the psychomotor choice of response.

4.1. The psychomotor response chosen will be activated through intact effectors.

5.1. Effector activity produces the response that is at an adaptive level, determined by the total functioning of the cognator subsystem.

6.1. The level of adaptive responses to internal and external stimuli will alter those internal and external stimuli. (Roy & McLeod, 1981, p. 65)

5

Theory of Adaptive Modes

The Theory of Adaptive Modes was developed in 1981 and has undergone substantial revision. The theory consists of four parts, each focusing on one of four adaptive modes: physiological, self-concept, role function, and interdependence. It is important to remember that each adaptive mode represents a grouping of behaviors that promote the individual's movement toward the general goals (survival, growth, reproduction, and mastery). A basic need has been identified in relation to each adaptive mode.

Physiological Mode

The basic human need within the physiological mode is for physiological integrity. Physiological wholeness (integrity) is "achieved by adapting to changes in physiological needs" (Andrews & Roy, 1991c, p. 58). The regulator coping mechanism is primarily responsible for attaining and maintaining this integrity. Five primary needs have been identified as necessary for physiological integrity: oxygen, nutrition, elimination, activity and rest, and protection. Other complex processes that influence regulator activities are the senses, fluids and electrolytes, neurological function, and endocrine function.

An adaptation problem in relation to the physiological need for protection would be pressure sores. The focal stimulus might be prolonged pressure over a bony area. Poor nutrition, incontinence, and edema would be examples of possible contextual stimuli. Residual stimuli might include the nurse's hunch that the way in which bed sheets are washed may contribute to the problem.

In Roy's Theory of Adaptive Modes, physiological propositions developed for the regulator mechanism were used to develop additional relational statements within the physiological adaptive mode (Roy & Roberts, 1981). An example of a hypothesis in the activity/rest need category initially generated from a regulator proposition is: "If the nurse helps the patient maintain muscle tone through proper exercising, the patient will experience fewer problems associated with immobility" (p. 90).

Self-Concept Mode

Self-concept is one of three psychosocial modes. The basic human need within this mode is psychic integrity, which means "people need to know who they are so that they can exist with a sense of unity" (Roy & Andrews, 1991, p. 267). A person's level of self-esteem reflects the self-concept. Thus nursing diagnoses indicating adaptation problems and indicators of positive adaptation with regard to self-esteem are commonly found in the self-concept mode. Self-concept is "the composite of beliefs and feelings that one holds about oneself at a given time, formed from perceptions particularly of others' reactions, and directing one's behavior" (Driever cited in Andrews, 1991a, p. 270). Self-concept has been categorized into physical self and personal self.

Physical self. Physical self is an "appraisal of one's physical attributes, appearance, functioning, sensation, sexuality, and wellness-illness status" (Buck, 1991a, p. 282). Physical self has been further divided into body sensation (how one feels about one's self) and body image (how one thinks one's body looks and how one feels about how one's body looks). An example of a disturbance in the body image component of the physical self might be verbalizations by an anorexic patient that she is fat and wants to lose 10 pounds within the next month. Other nursing diagnoses, identified by Buck (1991a), that indicate adaptation problems in the physical self are sexual dysfunction and rape trauma syndrome.

Personal self. Personal self is an "appraisal of one's own characteristics, expectations, values, and worth" (Andrews, 1991a, p. 270). Personal self has been subdivided into the moral-ethical-spiritual self, self-consistency, and self-ideal/self-expectancy.

The moral-ethical-spiritual self is the individual's morals and belief system. "I believe God will help me through this surgery" is an example of a verbalization behavior in a belief system. Spiritual distress is an example of a nursing diagnosis resulting from a disruption of the moral-ethical-spiritual self.

Self-consistency is the individual's actual performance and/or personality traits. "I'm usually a pretty even-tempered person" is a statement about an individual's self-consistency. Anxiety is a nursing diagnosis arising from an adaptation problem in this area of the self.

Self-ideal/self-expectancy is what one would like to do or become relative to one's capabilities. "I would like to finish high school by taking the GED" is a verbalization about self-ideal/self-expectancy. Powerlessness is a nursing diagnosis indicating a disruption in this part of the self-concept mode. Other adaptation problems in the self-concept mode have been identified by Buck (1991a, 1991b).

Self-Concept Mode Propositions

For the self-concept adaptive mode, separate propositions were developed using the same format as for the coping mechanisms. Figure 5.1 depicts the parts of the self-concept subsystem.

The propositions corresponding to Figure 5.1 are as follows:

1.1. The positive quality of social experience in the form of others' appraisals positively influences the level of feelings of adequacy.

1.2. Adequacy of role taking positively influences the quality of input in the form of social experience.

1.3. The number of social rewards positively influences the quality of social experience.

1.4. Negative feedback in the form of performance compared with ideals leads to corrections in levels of feelings of adequacy.

1.5. Conflicts in input in the form of varying appraisals positively influences the amount of self-concept confusion experienced.

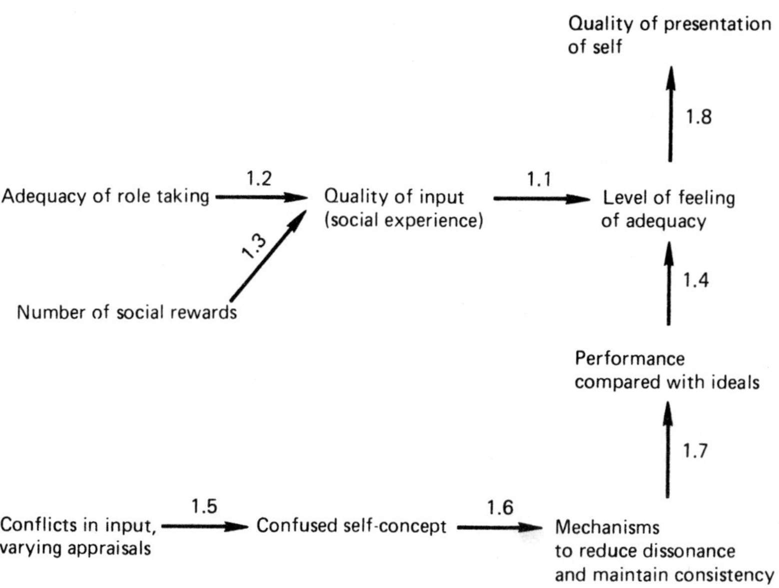

Figure 5.1. Linking of parts of the self-concept mode.
SOURCE: Roy & Roberts, 1981, p. 255. Reprinted by permission.

1.6. Confused self-concept leads to activation of mechanisms to reduce dissonance and maintain consistency.
1.7. Activity of mechanisms for reducing dissonance and maintaining consistency (e.g., choice) tends to lead to feelings of adequacy.
1.8. The level of feelings of adequacy positively influences the quality of presentation of self. (Roy & Roberts, 1981, p. 255)

Roy and Roberts (1981) give an example of a hypothesis generated from these propositions: "If the nurse helps the new mother to practice role taking, the mother will develop a higher level of feelings of adequacy" (p. 258).

Role Function Mode

The basic need in the role function adaptive mode is for social integrity. This means that people need to know who they are in relation to others so that they can act. All people have roles in society. With each role, there are expected behaviors (i.e., societal norms). A common nursing diagnosis of an adaptation problem in this mode would be altered role performance. Roles have been divided into primary, secondary, and tertiary.

Roles. The primary role is determined by the majority of behaviors that are engaged in by persons during specific periods in life; it is determined by age, gender, and developmental stage (e.g., 24-year-old female young adult.) Secondary roles are those that persons assume to complete tasks associated with the primary role and developmental stage. Secondary roles are normally achieved, and stable (e.g., wife, mother, and nurse). Tertiary roles are related primarily to the secondary roles, usually temporary, and are freely chosen. These roles represent ways in which people meet the obligations associated with their other roles. Hobbies also are included in tertiary roles. Examples of tertiary roles might be Scout leader, part-time graduate nursing student, and reader of mysteries. Some roles may change from tertiary to secondary; during an acute illness, for example, the person assumes a tertiary sick role; if the illness becomes chronic, the sick role becomes secondary.

Behaviors associated with roles. Instrumental and expressive behaviors are associated with each role. Instrumental behaviors are usually of a physical and long-term nature. The goal is role mastery for these action-oriented behaviors. An example of instrumental behavior in the secondary role is acquisition of psychomotor skills by nursing students. Expressive behaviors are usually of an emotional nature. They are expressions of feelings or attitudes for which the goal is direct or immediate feedback. The novice nurse discussing a patient care situation with an expert nurse is an example of expressive behavior.

Role performance requirements associated with roles. Four requirements for role performance are necessary before a person can engage in instrumental or expressive behaviors. In order to perform the role, there needs to be a consumer, a reward to the performer, facilities within which to perform the role, and cooperation. Questions that clarify the role requirements for instrumental behavior are as follows:

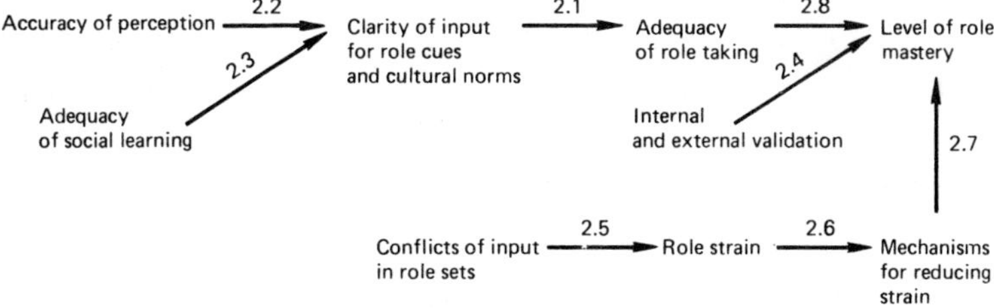

Figure 5.2. Linking of parts of the role function mode.
SOURCE: Roy & Roberts, 1981, p. 267. Reprinted by permission.

1. Consumer: Who or what benefits from the performance of the behavior?
2. Reward: What is the reward for the behavior?
3. Access to facilities/set of circumstances: What equipment, supplies, or tools are needed to perform the role?
4. Cooperation/collaboration: Is time allowed to perform the role behaviors?

Questions related to the role performance requirements for expressive behaviors are similar to those for instrumental behavior:

1. Consumer: Is there an appropriate and receptive person who will provide feedback?
2. Reward: Is there a network to provide feedback on role performance?
3. Access to facilities/set of circumstances: Do I have what I need to accomplish my task?
4. Collaboration/cooperation: Will the setting provide the circumstances and climate needed to fulfil the role? (Andrews, 1991b; Roy, 1984).

Role Function Mode Propositions

The relationships among concepts in the second psychosocial adaptive mode of role function are depicted in Figure 5.2, and, the numbered propositions correspond to the numbers in that figure.

2.1. The amount of clarity of input in the form of role cues and cultural norms positively influences the adequacy of role taking.
2.2. Accuracy of perception positively influences the clarity of input in the form of role cues and cultural norms.
2.3. Adequacy of social learning positively influences the clarity of input in the form of role cues and cultural norms.
2.4. Negative feedback in the form of internal and external validations leads to corrections in adequacy of role taking.
2.5. Conflicts in input in the form of conflicting role sets positively influence the amount of role strain experienced.
2.6. Role strain leads to activation of mechanisms for reducing role strain and for articulating role sets.
2.7. Activity of mechanisms for reducing role strain and for articulating role sets (e.g., choice) leads to adequacy of role taking.
2.8. The level of adequacy of role taking positively influences the level of role mastery. (Roy & Roberts, 1981, p. 267)

Again, Roy & Roberts (1981) offer an example of a hypothesis derived from the propositions: "If the nurse orients the patient to the sick role, the patient will perform at a higher level of role mastery in the sick role" (p. 270).

Interdependence Mode

Interdependence is a social adaptive mode. The basic need is affectional adequacy or the "feeling of security in nurturing relationships" (Tedrow, 1991, p. 386). Interdependence means "the close relationships of people that involve the willingness and ability to love, respect, and value others, and to accept and respond to love, respect, and value given by others" (p. 386). Servonsky and Tedrow (1991) identified loneliness as a common adaptation problem resulting from a disruption in this mode.

Behaviors. There are two types of behaviors within the interdependence adaptive mode: receptive and contributive. Receiving, taking-in, and/or assimilating nurturing behaviors offered by significant others or support systems are receptive behaviors. Contributive behaviors are those that give or supply nurturing to significant others or

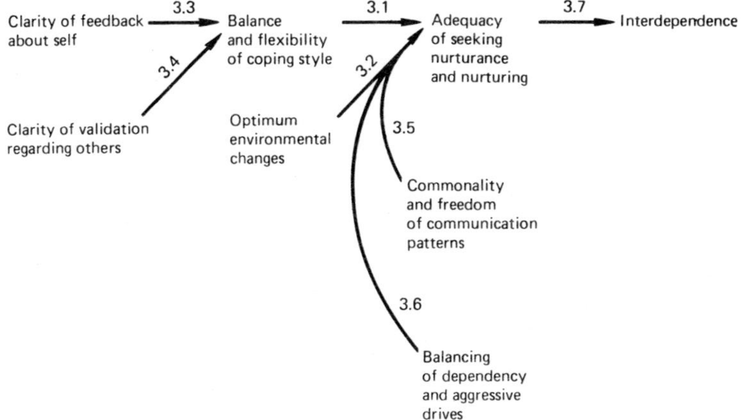

Figure 5.3. Linking of parts of the interdependence mode.
SOURCE: Roy & Roberts, 1981, p. 278. Reprinted by permission.

support systems. Significance may be assigned to another person or inherent in an interaction. Significant others have the most meaning or importance in a person's life. Support systems are continuing social collectives such as groups, organizations, and networks.

Interdependence Mode Propositions

Figure 5.3 depicts the schematic model that illustrates the propositions for this social mode, which are:

3.1. The balance and flexibility of coping style positively influence the adequacy of seeking nurturance and nurturing.
3.2. The optimum amount of environmental changes positively influences the adequacy of seeking nurturance and nurturing.
3.3. Clarity of feedback about self positively influences the balance and flexibility of coping style.
3.4. Clarity of validation regarding others positively influences the balance and flexibility of coping style.
3.5. Commonality and freedom of communication patterns positively influence the adequacy of seeking nurturance and nurturing.

3.6. The balancing of dependency and aggressive drives positively influences the adequacy of seeking nurturance and nurturing.
3.7. Adequacy of seeking nurturance and nurturing positively influences interdependence. (Roy & Roberts, 1981, p. 277)

An example of a hypothesis relevant for practice might be, "If the nurse provides the time and space for private family visits, the patient will demonstrate more appropriate attention-seeking behavior" (Roy & Roberts, 1981, p. 280).

More recently, Roy and Anway (1989) developed propositions for the Roy Adaptation Model to be applied to nursing administrative practice. Those propositions will not be listed here because it would be important to first understand the theory upon which the propositions are based.

6

Clinical Example

Many examples illustrating the use of the Roy Adaptation Model in various clinical settings have been published, some of which are described in the publications listed in the bibliography. Another example of how the RAM could be used in the clinical setting follows.

A woman in her mid-forties recently has been diagnosed with breast cancer. Having undergone a unilateral modified radical mastectomy, she is now faced with the prospect of chemotherapy. The nurse encounters the patient on her first post-operative day. The patient is alert and oriented, and denies pain or acute discomfort. The nurse observes facial tension, however, and a slight trembling of the patient's hands. The nurse asks the patient if she has had an opportunity to talk with the surgeon since her operation. The patient replies that the surgeon had visited her earlier that day and informed her that the medical oncologist would be in later to introduce herself and give an overview of the chemotherapy treatment. The patient states that, although she had been told she would also have "chemo" in addition to surgery, the news today was "final." She admits she had secretly hoped that the surgery "would be it." The tone of her voice is apprehensive. She expresses feelings of "being scared, jittery inside, and nervous." Having heard about the side effect of hair loss, she finds that upsetting. She has nice hair and has always been complimented on its color and body. She considers it one of her best features and so does her husband.

We can tentatively determine from a first-level assessment of the subjective and objective behaviors in the scenario that one nursing diagnosis is anxiety. The patient is experiencing a subjective awareness of information. In assessing the stimuli (second-level assessment), the nurse identifies the focal stimulus as concern over the chemotherapy side effect of hair loss. Contextual stimuli influencing how the patient deals with the focal stimulus are identified as the unknown experience of chemotherapy, the diagnosis of cancer, and concern over the husband's response to her hair loss. Residual stimuli would be the cultural norm of hair on the head of females and the general societal feeling about female appearance relative to hair. This patient's behaviors can be categorized in the physical self component of the self-concept adaptive mode. Her basic need is for psychic integrity, specifically with regard to body image.

Within the context of the discussion, both nurse and patient agree that a goal is to decrease patient anxiety. The nurse then selects interventions to manage the stimuli confronting the patient, thereby promoting adaptation of the patient to the environmental situation at hand (i.e., chemotherapy). The interventions include allowing the patient's verbalization; educating with regard to the chemotherapy, principally in terms of the power of drugs that destroy hair follicles in addition to cancer cells and the temporary nature of the hair loss; and reassuring with regard to the availability of attractive, well-fitting wigs that can be matched to her natural hair color and the fact that turbans are an "in" fashion item. The nurse and patient could also discuss how the husband could be involved in components of her care in a way that would be comfortable for both of them. The coping mechanism of cognator will assist the patient in processing information, learning about chemotherapy and wigs, selecting wigs and turbans, and talking with her husband about the imminent, yet tem- porary, hair loss. The effect from the activity of the patient's cognator coping mechanism will be observed principally in the body-image physical self component of the self-concept adaptive mode. Successful nursing interventions will result in a decrease or elimination of signs and symptoms of the patient's anxiety and an increase in necessary coping skills. Adaptive responses would include a more confident person with a positive body image regardless of the presence of a wig.

Research could be conducted on interventions used to promote adaptation of patients. The Tulman, Fawcett, Groblewski and Silverman (1990) article is one example of recent research using Roy's model.

7

Conclusion

The Roy Adaptation Model and its derived theories of Person as an Adaptive System and Adaptive Modes have been discussed in this volume in relation to origin, assumptions, key concepts, and propositions. Several schematic diagrams have been included to visually present major concepts and linkages within the theories. Finally, an example was presented of the use of Theory of Person as an Adaptive System in an application of the Roy model to medical-surgical patients in the hospital.

The Roy Adaptation Model has demonstrated utility in nursing practice, education, and, in a more limited fashion, research. A distinct advantage of the theories generated from Roy's model is their broad scope. They are applicable to all clinical settings. A limitation is the complexity of the regulator and cognator subsystems. The Theory of Adaptive Modes also has become increasingly complex since its initial development in 1981. The quantity and quality of the literature illustrating the Roy model are noteworthy and helpful to those desiring to learn more about the model and its relationship to the practice of nursing.

Glossary

Adaptation
"A process of responding positively to environmental changes in such a way as to decrease responses necessary to cope with the stimuli and increase sensitivity to respond to other stimuli" (Roy, 1984, p. 37); "the person's response to the environment which promotes the general goals of the person including survival, growth, reproduction, and mastery" (Roy & McLeod, 1981, p. 53); "a process of coping with stressors as well as the end state producted by this process" (Roy & McLeod, 1981, p. 57).

Adaptation level
"A changing point, influenced by the demands of the situation and the person's internal resources including capabilities, hopes, dreams, aspirations, motivations, and all that makes the person constantly move toward mastery" (Andrews & Roy, 1991a, p. 6); "focal, contextual, and residual stimuli pool to make up the person's adaptation level" (Andrews & Roy, 1991a, p. 10).

Adaptive
"The capacity to adjust effectively to changes in the environment and, in turn, affect the environment" (Andrews & Roy, 1991a, p. 6).

Adaptive behavior
See Adaptive responses.

Adaptive modes
"Ways of coping that show the activity of the regulator and cognator mechanisms" (Andrews & Roy, 1986, p. 7); "ways of categorizing the effects of cognator and regulator activity" (Roy, 1984, p. 22); "classification of ways of coping that manifest regulator and cognator activity, that is, physiologic, self-concept, role function, and interdependence" (Roy, 1984, p. 28); "provide the particular form or manifestation of cognator and regulator activity" (Roy & Roberts, 1981, p. 43, 67); "effectors of adaptation" (Roy & Roberts, 1981, pp. 43, 67).

Adaptive responses
"Promote the integrity of the person in terms of the goals of adaptation: survival, growth, reproduction, and mastery" (Andrews & Roy, 1991a, p. 12).

Adaptive zone
"Range of coping" (Andrews & Roy, 1986, p. 31); "stimulation [within the zone] will lead to a positive or adaptive response; stimuli that fall outside the zone lead to negative or ineffective responses" (Roy, 1984, p. 37).

Behavior
"Responses of the adaptive system" (Andrews & Roy, 1991a, p. 12); "actions and reactions under specified circumstances" (Andrews & Roy, 1986, p. 32).

Client of nursing
"A person, a family, a group, a community, or society" (Roy & Roberts, 1981, p. 42).

Cognator
Mechanism that "responds through four cognitive-emotive channels: perception and information processing, learning, judgment, and emotion" (Andrews & Roy, 1991a, p. 14); "involves the psychological processes for dealing cognitively and emotionally with the changing environment" (Roy, 1984, p. 22); one of two "ways or methods of adapting or coping" (Roy & McLeod, 1981, p. 66).

Contextual stimuli
"All the environmental factors that present to the person from within or without, but which are not the center of the person's attention and/or energy" (Andrews & Roy, 1991a, p. 9); "all other stimuli present, either within persons as their internal condition or coming as

input from the environment" (Roy, 1984, p. 37); "all other stimuli present that contribute to the behavior caused or precipitated by the focal stimulus" (Roy & Roberts, 1984, p. 43); "all other stimuli present in the situation of the stressor" (Roy & McLeod, 1981, p. 55); a mediating factor that contributes to the effect of the stressor (focal stimulus) (Roy & McLeod, 1981, p. 55).

Coping
"Routine, accustomed patterns of behavior to deal with daily situations as well as the production of new ways of behaving when drastic changes defy the familiar responses" (Roy & McLeod, 1981, p. 56); "operating to produce adaptive responses" (Roy & McLeod, 1981, p. 56).

Coping mechanism
"Innate or acquired ways of responding to the changing environment" (Andrews & Roy, 1991a, p. 13).

Innate: "genetically determined or common to a species"; "automatic process";

Acquired: "developed through processes such as learning" (Andrews & Roy, 1991a, p. 13).

Environment
"All conditions, circumstances, and influences that surround and affect the development and behavior of the person" (Andrews & Roy, 1991a, p. 18).

First-level assessment
"Gathering data about behavior in each adaptive mode by skillful observation, accurate measurement of responses, and communicative interviewing" (Roy, 1984, p. 43).

Focal stimulus
"The internal or external stimulus most immediately confronting the person; the object or event that attracts one's attention" (Andrews & Roy, 1991a, p. 8); "degree of change that precipitates adaptive behavior; stimulus most immediately confronting the person, the one to which he must make an adaptive response; stressor" (Roy & McLeod, 1981, p. 55).

Goal of nursing
"Promotion of adaptation in each of the four modes, thereby contributing to the person's health, quality of life, and dying with dignity" (Andrews & Roy, 1991a, p. 20); "to promote patient adaptation in regard to the four [adaptive] modes" (Roy & Roberts, 1981, p. 44).

Health
"A state and a process of being and becoming an integrated and whole person . . . a reflection of adaptation" (Andrews & Roy, 1991a, p. 19).

Holistic
"Pertains to the idea that the human system functions as a whole and is more than the mere sum of its parts" (Andrews & Roy, 1991a, p. 6).

Humanism
"Recognizes the person and subjective dimensions of human experience as central to knowing and to valuing" (Roy, 1988, p. 29).

Ineffective response
Behavior that "does not promote integrity nor contribute to the goals of adaptation" (Andrews & Roy, 1991a, p. 12); "behavior that does not lead to [goal attainment] or that disrupts the integrity of the individual" (Roy & McLeod, 1981, p. 57).

Integrity
"Degree of wholeness achieved by adapting to changes in needs" (Andrews & Roy, 1991c, p. 59).

Interdependence
"The close relationships of people that involve the willingness and ability to love, respect, and value others, and to accept and respond to love, respect, and value given by others" (Tedrow, 1991, p. 386).

Living system
"A whole made up of parts or subsystems that function as a unity for some purpose" (Roy & McLeod, 1981, p. 53).

Nursing activities
"Assess behavior and factors that influence adaptation level and intervene by managing the focal, contextual, and residual stimuli" (Roy, 1984, p. 13); nursing process.

Nursing diagnosis
"Judgment process resulting in a statement conveying the person's adaptation status" (Andrews & Roy, 1991b, p. 37); "interpretation of assessment data stated as a summary label for one mode, as a statement of the behaviors within one mode, with the most relevant influencing factors, or as a label that summarizes a behavioral pattern with more than one mode being affected by the same stimuli" (Roy, 1984, p. 43).

Nursing intervention
Management of stimuli that "involves altering, increasing, decreasing, removing, or maintaining" focal, contextual, and residual stimuli (Andrews & Roy, 1991b, p. 44); "selection and carrying out of an approach to change or stabilize adaptation by managing stimuli" (Roy, 1984, p. 43); "carried out in the context of the nursing process" (Roy & Roberts, 1981, p. 46).

Person
"Holistic adaptive system" (Andrews & Roy, 1991a, p. 6); "an adaptive system with cognator and regulator acting to maintain adaptation in regard to the four adaptive modes" (Roy & Roberts, 1981, pp. 44, 48); biopsychosocial being in constant interaction with a changing environment (Roy, 1980).

Regulator
"Responds automatically through neural, chemical, and endocrine coping processes" (Andrews & Roy, 1991a, p. 14).

Residual stimuli
Factors "having an indeterminate effect on the person's behavior; their effect has not or cannot be validated" (Andrews & Roy, 1991b, p. 35); "environmental factors within or [outside] the person whose effects in the current situation are unclear, possible, yet uncertain, influencing stimuli" (Andrews & Roy, 1986, p. 29); includes beliefs, attitudes, experience, or traits (Roy, 1984); mediating factors that contribute to the effect of the stressor (focal stimulus); "presumed to effect the current situation, although this effect cannot be validated or measured" (Roy & McLeod, 1981, p. 56).

Second-level assessment
"Identification of the focal, contextual, and residual factors that influence the person" (Roy, 1984, p. 43).

Self-concept
"Composite of beliefs and feelings that one holds about oneself at a given time, formed from perceptions particularly of others' reactions, and directing one's behavior" (Driever cited in Andrews, 1991a, p. 270).

Significant other
"The individual to whom the most meaning or importance is given. It is a person who is loved, respected, and valued; and who, in turn, loves, respects, and values the other to a degree greater than in all other relationships" (Tedrow, 1991, p. 386).

Stimuli
"That which provokes a response" (Andrews & Roy, 1991b, p. 33); "inputs for the person . . . [that] come from the [outside] environment (external stimuli) and internally from the self (internal stimuli)" (Andrews & Roy, 1986, p. 21).

Stressor
"Demand for an adaptive response" (Roy & McLeod, 1981, p. 55); focal stimuli mediated by contextual and residual factors (Roy & McLeod, 1981).

Veritivity
"A principle of human nature that affirms a common purposefulness of human existence" (Roy, 1988, p. 30).

References

Andrews, H. A. (1991a). Overview of the self-concept mode. In C. Roy & H. A. Andrews, *The Roy adaptation model: The definitive statement* (pp. 269-279). Norwalk, CT: Appleton & Lange.

Andrews, H. A. (1991b). Overview of the role function mode. In C. Roy & H. A. Andrews, *The Roy adaptation model: The definitive statement* (pp. 347-361). Norwalk, CT: Appleton & Lange.

Andrews, H. A., & Roy, C. (1986). *Essentials of the Roy adaptation model.* Norwalk, CT: Appleton-Century-Crofts.

Andrews, H. A., & Roy, C. (1991a). Essentials of the Roy adaptation model. In C. Roy & H. A. Andrews, *The Roy adaptation model: The definitive statement* (pp. 3-25). Norwalk, CT: Appleton & Lange.

Andrews, H. A., & Roy, C. (1991b). The nursing process according to the Roy adaptation model. In C. Roy & H. A. Andrews, *The Roy adaptation model: The definitive statement* (pp. 27-54). Norwalk, CT: Appleton & Lange.

Andrews, H. A., & Roy, C. (1991c). Overview of the physiological mode. In C. Roy & H. A. Andrews, *The Roy adaptation model: The definitive statement* (pp. 57-66). Norwalk, CT: Appleton & Lange.

Buck, M. (1991a). The physical self. In C. Roy & H. A. Andrews, *The Roy adaptation model: The definitive statement* (pp. 281-310). Norwalk, CT: Appleton & Lange.

Buck, M. (1991b). The personal self. In C. Roy & H. A. Andrews, *The Roy adaptation model: The definitive statement* (pp. 311-355). Norwalk, CT: Appleton & Lange.

Roy, C. (1971). Adaptation: A basis for nursing practice. *Nursing Outlook, 19,* 254-257.

Roy, C. (1980). The Roy adaptation model. In J. P. Riehl & C. Roy (Eds.), *Conceptual models for nursing practice* (2nd ed., pp. 179-192). New York: Appleton-Century-Crofts.

Roy, C. (1984). *Introduction to nursing: An adaptation model* (2nd ed.). Englewood Cliffs, NJ: Prentice-Hall.

Roy, C. (1988). An explication of the philosophical assumptions of the Roy adaptation mode. *Nursing Science Quarterly, 1*(1), 26-34.

Roy, C. (1990). Strengthening the Roy adaptation model through conceptual clarification: Response. *Nursing Science Quarterly,* 3(2), 64-66.

Roy, C., & Andrews, H. A. (1991). *The Roy adaptation model: The definitive statement.* Norwalk, CT: Appleton & Lange.

Roy, C., & Anway, J. (1989). Roy's adaptation model: Theories for nursing administration. In B. Henry, C. Arndt, M. Di Vincenti, & A. Marriner-Tomey (Eds.), *Dimensions of nursing administration: Theory, research, education, practice* (pp. 75-88). Boston: Blackwell Scientific.

Roy, C., & McLeod, D. (1981). Theory of person as an adaptive system. In C. Roy & S. L. Roberts, *Theory construction in nursing: An adaptation model* (pp. 49-69). Englewood Cliffs, NJ: Prentice-Hall.

Roy, C., & Roberts, S. L. (1981). *Theory construction in nursing: An adaptation model.* Englewood Cliffs, NJ: Prentice-Hall.

Sato, M. K. (1984). Major factors influencing adaptation. In C. Roy, *Introduction to nursing: An adaptation model* (2nd ed., pp. 64-87). Englewood Cliffs, NJ: Prentice-Hall.

Servonsky, J., & Tedrow, M. P. (1991). Separation anxiety and loneliness. In C. Roy & H. A. Andrews, *The Roy adaptation model: The definitive statement* (pp. 405-422). Norwalk, CT: Appleton & Lange.

Tedrow, M. P. (1991). Overview of the interdependence mode. In C. Roy & H. A. Andrews, *The Roy adaptation model: The definitive statement* (pp. 385-403). Norwalk, CT: Appleton & Lange.

Tulman, L., Fawcett, J., Groblewski, L., & Silverman, L. (1990). Changes in functional status after childbirth. *Nursing Research, 39,* 70-75.

Bibliography

Theory

Andrews, H. A., & Roy, C. (1986). *Essentials of the Roy adaptation model.* Norwalk, CT: Appleton-Century-Crofts.

Blue, C. L., Brubaker, K. M., Fine, J. M., Kirsch, M. J., Papazian, K. R., & Riester, C. M. (1989). Sister Callista Roy: Adaptation model. In A. Marriner-Tomey (Ed.), *Nursing theorists and their work* (2nd ed., pp. 325-411). St. Louis: C. V. Mosby.

Buck, M. H. (1984). Self-concept: Theory and development. In C. Roy, *Introduction to nursing: An adaptation model* (2nd ed., pp. 255-283). Englewood Cliffs, NJ: Prentice-Hall.

Chinn, P. L., & Kramer, M. K. (1991). *Theory and nursing: A systematic approach* (3rd ed., p. 187). St. Louis: C. V. Mosby.

DeFeo, D. J. (1990). Change: A central concern of nursing. *Nursing Science Quarterly, 3*, 88-94.

Galbreath, J. G. (1990). Sister Callista Roy. In J. B. George, *Nursing theories: The base for professional nursing practice* (3rd ed.). Norwalk, CT: Appleton & Lange.

Nuwayhid, K. A. (1984). Role function: Theory and development. In C. Roy, *Introduction to nursing: An adaptation model* (2nd ed., pp. 284-305). Englewood Cliffs, NJ: Prentice-Hall.

Roy, C. (1970). Adaptation: A conceptual framework for nursing. *Nursing Outlook, 18*(3), 42-45.

Roy, C. (1971). Adaptation: A basis for nursing practice. *Nursing Outlook, 19*, 254-257.

Roy, C. (1983). Roy adaptation model. In I. W. Clements & F. B. Roberts (Eds.), *Family health: A theoretical approach to nursing care* (pp. 255-277). New York: Wiley.

Roy, C. (1984). *Introduction to nursing: An adaptation model* (2nd ed.). Englewood Cliffs, NJ: Prentice-Hall.

Roy, C. (1987). Roy's adaptation model. In R. R. Parse (Ed.), *Nursing science: Major paradigms, theories, and critiques* (pp. 35-45). Philadelphia: W. B. Saunders.

Roy, C. (1988). An explication of the philosophical assumptions of the Roy adaptation model. *Nursing Science Quarterly, 1,* 26-34.

Roy, C. (1989). The Roy adaptation model. In J. P. Riehl-Sisca (Ed.), *Conceptual models for nursing practice* (3rd ed., pp. 105-114). Norwalk, CT: Appleton & Lange.

Roy, C., & Andrews, H. A. (1991). *The Roy adaptation model: The definitive statement.* Norwalk, CT: Appleton & Lange.

Roy, C., & McLeod, D. (1981). Theory of person as an adaptive system. In C. Roy & S. L. Roberts, *Theory construction in nursing: An adaptation model* (pp. 49-69). Englewood Cliffs, NJ: Prentice-Hall.

Roy, C., & Roberts, S. L. (1981). *Theory construction in nursing: An adaptation model.* Englewood Cliffs, NJ: Prentice-Hall.

Sato, M. K. (1984). Major factors influencing adaptation. In C. Roy, *Introduction to nursing: An adaptation model* (2nd ed., pp. 64-87). Englewood Cliffs, NJ: Prentice-Hall.

Tedrow, M. P. (1984). Interdependence: Theory and development. In C. Roy, *Introduction to nursing: An adaptation model* (2nd ed., pp. 306-322). Englewood Cliffs, NJ: Prentice-Hall.

Tiedeman, M. E. (1989). The Roy adaptation model. In J. Fitzpatrick & A. Whall, *Conceptual models of nursing: Analysis and application* (2nd ed., pp. 185-204). Bowie, MD: Brady.

Analysis and Evaluation of the Roy Adaptation Model

Artinian, N. T. (1990). Strengthening the Roy adaptation model through conceptual clarification: Commentary. *Nursing Science Quarterly, 3,* 60-64.

Fawcett, J. (1989). Roy's adaptation model. In J. Fawcett, *Analysis and evaluation of conceptual models of nursing* (2nd ed., pp. 307-353). Philadelphia: F. A. Davis.

Giger, J. N. (1990). Nightingale and Roy: A comparison of nursing models. *Today's OR Nurse, 12*(4), 25-28, 30-33.

Huch, M. H. (1987). A critique of the Roy adaptation model. In R. R. Parse (Ed.), *Nursing science: Major paradigms, theories, and critiques* (pp. 47-66). Philadelphia: W. B. Saunders.

Mastal, M. F., & Hammond, H. (1980). Analysis and expansion of the Roy adaptation model: A contribution to holistic nursing. *Advances in Nursing Science, 2*(4), 71-81.

Meleis, A. I. (1985). Sister Callista Roy. In A. I. Meleis, *Theoretical nursing: Development and progress* (pp. 206-218). Philadelphia: J. B. Lippincott.

Roy, C. (1990). Strengthening the Roy adaptation model through conceptual clarification: Response. *Nursing Science Quarterly, 3,* 64-66.

Extensions of the Roy Adaptation Model to Groups

DiIorio, C. K. (1989). Application of the Roy model to nursing administration. In B. Henry, C. Arndt, M. Di Vincenti, & A. Marriner-Tomey, *Dimensions of nursing administration: Theory, research, education, practice* (pp. 89-104). Boston: Blackwell Scientific.

Hanchett, E. S. (1988). Callista Roy—Focus: Adaptive systems. In E. S. Hanchett, *Nursing frameworks and community as client: Bridging the gap* (pp. 49-78). Norwalk, CT: Appleton & Lange.

Hanchett, E. S. (1990). Nursing models and community as client. *Nursing Science Quarterly, 3*, 67-72.

Roy, C. (1983a). Analysis and application of the Roy adaptation model. In I. W. Clements & F. B. Roberts (Eds.), *Family health: A theoretical approach to nursing care* (pp. 298-303). New York: Wiley.

Roy, C. (1983b). Analysis and application of the Roy adaptation model. In I. W. Clements & F. B. Roberts (Eds.), *Family health: A theoretical approach to nursing care* (pp. 375-378). New York: Wiley.

Roy, C., & Anway, J. (1989). Roy's adaptation model: Theories for nursing administration. In B. Henry, C. Arndt, M. Di Vincenti, & A. Marriner-Tomey (Eds.), *Dimensions of nursing administration: Theory, research, education, practice* (pp. 75-88). Boston: Blackwell Scientific.

Applications to Practice and Research

Barnfather, J. S., Swain, M. A. P., & Erickson, H. C. (1989). Evaluation of two assessment techniques for adaptation to stress. *Nursing Science Quarterly, 2*, 172-182.

Calvert, M. M. (1989). Human-pet interaction and loneliness: A test of concepts from Roy's adaptation model. *Nursing Science Quarterly, 2*, 194-202.

DiMaria, R. A. (1989). Posttrauma responses: Potential for nursing. *Journal of Advanced Medical Surgical Nursing, 2*(1), 41-48.

Downey, C. (1974). Adaptation nursing applied to an obstetric patient. In J. P. Riehl & C. Roy (Eds.), *Conceptual models for nursing practice* (pp. 151-159). New York: Appleton-Century-Crofts.

Farkas, L. (1981). Adaptation problems with nursing home application for elderly persons: An application of the Roy adaptation nursing model. *Journal of Advanced Nursing, 6*, 363-368.

Fawcett, J. (1981a). Assessing and understanding the cesarean father. In C. F. Kehoe (Ed.), *The cesarean experience: Theoretical and clinical perspectives for nurses*. New York: Appleton-Century-Crofts.

Fawcett, J. (1981b). Needs of cesarean birth parents. *Journal of Obstetric, Gynecologic, and Neonatal Nursing, 10*, 371-376.

Fawcett, J., & Tulman, L. (1990). Building a programme of research from the Roy adaptation model of nursing. *Journal of Advanced Nursing, 15*, 720-725.

Galligan, A. C. (1979). Using Roy's concept of adaptation to care for young children. *The American Journal of Maternal Child Nursing, 4*(1), 24-28.

Giger, J. A., Bower, C. A., & Miller, S. W. (1987). Roy adaptation model: ICU adaptation model: ICU application. *Dimensions of Critical Care Nursing, 6*, 215-224.

Gordon, J. (1974). Nursing assessment and care plan for a cardiac patient. In J. P. Riehl & C. Roy (Eds.), *Conceptual models for nursing practice* (pp. 144-150). New York: Appleton-Century-Crofts.

Hoch, C. C. (1987). Assessing delivery of nursing care. *Journal of Gerontological Nursing, 13,* 10-17.

Janelli, L. M. (1980). Utilizing Roy's adaptation model from a gerontological perspective. *Journal of Gerontological Nursing, 6,* 140-150.

Kehoe, C. F. (1981). Identifying the nursing needs of the postpartum cesarean mother. In C. F. Kehoe (Ed.), *The cesarean experience: Theoretical and clinical perspectives for nurses.* New York: Appleton-Century-Crofts.

Leuze, M., & McKenzie, J. (1987). Preoperative assessment: Using the Roy adaptation model. *AORN Journal, 46,* 1122-1134.

Limandri, B. J. (1986). Research and practice with abused women: Use of the Roy adaptation model as an explanatory framework. *Advances in Nursing Science, 8*(4), 52-61.

Logan, M. (1990). The Roy adaptation model: Are nursing diagnoses amenable to independent nurse functions? *Journal of Advanced Nursing, 15,* 468-470.

Mastal, M., Hammond, H., & Roberts. M. (1982). Theory into hospital practice: A pilot implementation. *The Journal of Nursing Administration, 12*(6), 9-15.

Mitchell, G. J., & Pilkington, B. (1990). Theoretical approaches in nursing practice: A comparison of Roy and Parse. *Nursing Science Quarterly, 3,* 88-94.

Norris, S., Campbell, L., & Brenkert, S. (1982). Nursing procedures and alternations in transcutaneous oxygen tension in premature infants. *Nursing Research, 31,* 330-336.

Pollock, S. E., Christian, B. J., & Sands, D. (1990). Responses to chronic illness: Analysis of psychological and physiological adaptation. *Nursing Research, 39,* 300-304.

Randell, B., Tedrow, M. P., & Van Landingham, J. (1982). *Adaptation nursing: The Roy conceptual model applied.* St. Louis: C. V. Mosby.

Roy, C. (1967). Role cues and mothers of hospitalized children. *Nursing Research, 16,* 178-182.

Roy, C. (1971). Adaptation: A basis for nursing practice. *Nursing Outlook, 19,* 254-257.

Roy, C. (1975). A diagnostic classification system for nursing. *Nursing Outlook, 23,* 90-94.

Silva, M. C. (1987). Needs of spouses of surgical patients: A conceptualization within the Roy adaptation model. *Scholarly Inquiry for Nursing Practice: An International Journal, 1*(1), 29-44.

Schmitz, M. (1980). The Roy adaptation model: Application in a community setting. In J. P. Riehl & C. Roy (Eds.), *Conceptual models for nursing practice* (2nd ed., pp. 193-206). New York: Appleton-Century-Crofts.

Smith, M. C. (1988). Roy's adaptation model in practice. *Nursing Science Quarterly, 1,* 97-98.

Starn, J., & Niederhauser, V. (1990). An MCN model for nursing diagnosis to focus intervention. *MCN, 15,* 180-183.

Starr, S. L. (1980). Adaptation applied to the dying patient. In J. P. Riehl & C. Roy (Eds.), *Conceptual models for nursing practice* (2nd ed., pp. 189-192). New York: Appleton-Century-Crofts.

Tulman, L., & Fawcett, J. (1990a). A framework for studying functional status after diagnosis of breast cancer. *Cancer Nursing, 13,* 95-99.

Tulman, L. & Fawcett, J. (1990b). Functional status during pregnancy and the postpartum: A framework for research. *Image, 22,* 191-194.

Tulman, L., Fawcett, J., Groblewski, L., & Silverman, L. (1990). Changes in functional status after childbirth. *Nursing Research, 39,* 70-75.

Wagner, P. (1976). Testing the adaptation model in practice. *Nursing Outlook, 24,* 682-685.

Applications to Education

Brower, H. T. F., & Baker, B. J. (1976). The Roy adaptation model: Using the adaptation model in a practitioner curriculum. *Nursing Outlook, 24,* 686-689.

Camooso, C., Green, M., & Reilly, P. (1981). Students' adaptation according to Roy. *Nursing Outlook, 29,* 57-65.

Morales-Mann, E. T., & Logan, M. (1990). Implementing the Roy model: Challenges for nurse educators. *Journal of Advanced Nursing, 15,* 720-725.

Roy, C. (1973). Adaptation: Implications for curriculum change. *Nursing Outlook, 21,* 163-165.

Roy, C. (1975). Adaptation: Implications for curriculum change. *Nursing Outlook, 23,* 90-94.

Roy, C. (1979). Relating nursing theory to education: A new era. *Nurse Educator,* 4(2), 16-20.

About the Author

Louette R. Johnson Lutjens, PhD, RN, is Associate Professor of Nursing at Grand Valley State University in Allendale, Michigan. She received her Doctor of Philosophy in Nursing degree in 1990 from Wayne State University in Detroit, Michigan. Her research interests include nursing administrative issues related to nursing diagnosis, interventions, and aggregate patient outcomes and theory development and testing.